CBD Oil and Hemp Oil

The Amazing CBD Oil Benefits for Pain, Anxiety, and Other CBD Oil Benefits for Overall Health

Erica Dube

Copyright © 2017 by Erica Dube

All rights reserved.

Publisher's Disclaimer

This book is for informational purposes only. Each individual's situation is unique. Use proper discretion and consult with a health care practitioner before putting the strategies, diets, or techniques described in this book. The authors and publisher disclaim responsibility for all adverse effects that may result from using or applying the information in this book.

Contents

Introduction	1
Chapter 1 History Benefits Of Cbd Oil	6
Chapter 2 Side Effects, Safety, And Cbd Oil Legality	17
Chapter 3 Cbd Oil For Pain	23
Chapter 4 Cbd Oil For Anxiety	31
Chapter 5 Cbd Oil And Parkinson's Disease	38
Chapter 6 Cbd Oil For Add And Adhd	45
Chapter 7 Cbd Oil And Alzheimer's	49
Chapter 8 Fibromyalgia And Cbd	54
Chapter 9 Buying Cbd Oil	59
Chapter 10 Growing Cannabis Plants And Making Cbd Oil	66
Chapter 11 Cancer, Cbd And Hemp Oils	76
Chapter 12 Hemp Oil	83
Chapter 13 The Difference Between Hemp, Cannabis, And More	96
Chapter 14 Rick Simpson Oil	103

Introduction

People across the world are prejudiced against the use of cannabis. Due to this, they are often not interested in learning about the research conducted to understand the benefits of cannabis. Most people are worried about how this plant could be abused as a drug. They often question whether CBD oil or hemp oil can help people deal with a variety of medical conditions. Thorough research has been conducted to understand how these oils work on the human body. This research gives rise to the following question: should CBD oil and hemp oil be legalized for medicinal use? Could the legalization lead to people giving into substance abuse? These questions cannot be answered yet. However, studies have been conducted recently have brought to light the different ways these chemicals function on the body.

It is unfortunate that the one thing people often talk about is whether or not cannabis should be legalized. People avoid discussing the medicinal properties of cannabis and do not spend any time trying to understand the benefits of those properties on the human body. This book attempts to bring the benefits of using cannabis and CBD oil to the forefront of discussion and talks about how these oils affect our bodies.

A lot of people have heard more about CBD oil and hemp oil, but they are not quite sure what the difference between the two is. Hemp products have been available for many years. It can be used in cooking products, cosmetic products, and everything in between. However, whenever people began to focus on the effects that cannabis had on health issues, people quickly got confused at what the difference between hemp oil and CBD oil was.

Hemp is typically used for industrial purposes. Hemp comes from a plant that tends to grow tall and has less than 0.3% THC content. Hemp is legal to use and to sell.

CBD oil is pulled from the leaves and flowers of a cannabis plant. Even though hemp and Sativa and even Indica are tied under the cannabis name, they are not going to have the same effects that CBD oil is going to have.

Hemp Oil

Hemp can be made by crushing hemp seeds that contain a low CBD count. The oil is usually used for topical applications such as shampoo, lotion, and soap. Hemp seeds can be eaten too as they are or they can be added and used as protein in health food supplements.

CBD Oil

While hemp oil is made from seeds that come from a hemp plant, CBD oil is going to come from the flowers of a cannabis plant and sometimes even the leaves and stalks of the plant so that there is a wider range of cannabinoids included in the oil from the plant.

The rich oil extracts from CBD is going to have a low THC content. In case you do not know, CBD stands for cannabidiol. And, this oil is not psychoactive like many people would think since it's made from the cannabis plant. There has been a lot of research conducted which show that CBD oil is beneficial to a person's health.

Unlike hemp oil, CBD oil can be used topically as well as internally.

Both hemp and CBD oil can be used to enrich your health. However, it is important for you to know that CBD oil is often used to heal a person. The higher the CBD count in your oil, the more effective it will be whenever you use it.

Throughout this book, you are going to learn the benefits that you are going to get from CBD oil and hemp oil. There are some important pieces of information that you are going to need to know to use CBD oil and hemp oil which you will learn right here!

Chapter 1

History Benefits of CBD Oil

CBD oil is most popular among people who suffer from stress, depression, chronic pain, sleep disorders, inflammation, anxiety, insomnia, and many other conditions. People often come across CBD oil when they are in too much pain and have exhausted all other traditional medication.

History of CBD Oil

CBD or Cannabidiol has gained popularity in recent years as people are trying to understand the benefits of CBD oil on the human body if it were used as a supplement or substitute. When you come across the multiple studies and research papers written on CBD oil, you may assume that CBD oil is a recent discovery. This is untrue since CBD oil has been used for quite some time. It is only the extraction of CBD and its packaging that have been discovered recently.

In early 2010, scientists and the general public were eager to see the effects that CBD oil has on the human body. It was observed that the oil helped prevent or cure certain life-threatening ailments and had a stronger effect on children. A classic example of this would be the story of Cash Hyde. Cash was diagnosed with brain cancer at the tender age of 20 months. His parents had tried every treatment that was available in the medical world, but Cash showed no improvement, and the tumor in his brain became inoperable. The family had exhausted every possible treatment available including 30 rounds of chemo, Ketamine, Methadone, and Morphine.

Cash's father, Mike, then administered a treatment on Cash that is often frowned upon. He gave his son an extract of Cannabis, which had a higher concentration of CBD in it. After using this extract for a small period, the tumor had shrunk in size. Mike was applauded by the medical community and had given a number of interviews that helped shed some light on the medicinal benefits of CBD oil. Cash lived a healthy life for two and a half years after until the cancer came back. His parents were unable to treat him using CBD oil since the state of Montana made it difficult to access the oil.

Another medical miracle, which received a lot of national press, took place in the year 2013. A three-year-old from Colorado, Charlotte Figi, suffered from epilepsy and had uncontrollable seizures every week. Her parents had tried every treatment that was available to them to help control these seizures. They were devastated when none of the treatments available to them worked on their child. It was when they watched a documentary on how medical marijuana could be used to treat epilepsy that they decided to use it on their daughter. There was a medical dispensary in California where certain strands of marijuana, with a higher concentration of CBD, were tested to understand the medicinal benefits. This dispensary made a public assertion that CBD oil could indeed be used to treat a number of medical disorders. Charlotte's parents then administered CBD oil on her; they were elated to see that she stopped having multiple seizures every week and the intensity of those seizures decreased. This incident gained immense popularity in 2013.

These few incidents and other scientific studies show that CBD oil helps to enhance a person's well being. The incidents mentioned above laid the groundwork, which made the world realize that CBD oil could be used as a medicine to treat a number of ailments. It is for this reason alone that CBD oil has now been legalized in a number of states.

Benefits of CBD Oil

In this section, we are going to go over some of the main benefits of using CBD oil. I'll go into more depth in later chapters as well.

Improves Appetite

The body processes CBD oil to control appetite. Your body releases hormones that help control your hunger and help you feel satiated after consuming a meal. It is only when these hormones are at balance, will you be able to maintain a healthy appetite. This balance is particularly helpful when it comes to times of serious illness, injury, or if you have had surgery. Most illnesses and medical conditions suppress appetite due to mostly prescription medication.

Skin Care

CBD oil can be used to improve the appearance of your skin especially if you have acne or eczema. You can apply diluted CBD oil or the oil in its pure form on your skin depending on how severe the affliction is. Because CBD oil has powerful anti-inflammatory properties, it can also soothe redness, swollen, and itchy areas of your skin.

Relieves Pain

One of the biggest arguments for CBD oil is that it can help those who suffer from chronic pain caused either by a backache or even cancer. CBD oil disrupts the activity of the pain receptors in your body and causes neurotransmitters to release such hormones like dopamine and serotonin to ease the pain.

Combats Alzheimer's disease

CBD oil can be used effectively to treat Alzheimer's disease. A number of studies have been conducted on the usage of CBD oil, which shows that those who use CBD oil have a lower probability of getting neurodegenerative diseases. These studies conclude that CBD oil helps control the development of certain traits of the disorder in the patient. For example, one such study concluded that CBD helped in the controlling the development of the loss of social recognition, which prevented the patient from forgetting faces.

Reduces Anxiety

While some people tend to say that marijuana makes them paranoid, CBD oil can reduce those feelings of anxiety by increasing positive hormones and neurotransmitters to release in the body.

Patients suffering from chronic anxiety are usually not prescribed CBD Oil since there are a lot of misconceptions about the benefits of the oil.

Many studies were conducted to understand the effect of CBD oil on certain anxiety disorders. Some of the conditions that can be controlled using CBD oil are listed below:

- Social Anxiety disorder
- Panic disorder
- Obsessive Compulsive disorder
- Post-traumatic Stress disorder
- General Anxiety disorder

Most of the drugs that are administered to the patients often have side effects. CBD oil does not have drastic side effects if it is used in moderation. There are a number of studies that show how CBD oil can be used as an alternative to the conventional drugs. However, further research is necessary to understand how CBD oil can be used effectively.

Lowers Inflammation

Some people have reported that when it comes to inflammation, they can only find relief with CBD oil. CBD oil can reduce inflammation caused by rheumatoid arthritis and joint disorders as well as other disorders that cause pain and inflammation.

Treats Epilepsy

Only highly concentrated doses of the oil have been known to treat epilepsy successfully. There has also been some success in using CBD oil to prevent epilepsy. This offers new hope to those who suffer from this seizure-inducing condition.

Extensive research has been conducted to see how CBD oil can be used to treat epilepsy and neuropsychiatric disorders. A recent study that was posted in "Epilepsia" stated that CBD oil is of little or no risk to people who are suffering from epilepsy. The oil has anti-seizure properties that help to lessen the intensity of seizures and also the number of seizures. Further research has stated that CBD oil could also contribute to treating a number of other neurological disorders related to epilepsy-like neuronal injury, neurodegeneration, and other psychiatric disorders. CBD can also be used as a treatment for schizophrenia as opposed to the antipsychotic drugs that are currently in use (these have adverse side effects on the person).

Prevents Cancer

Over the past decade, a number of studies were conducted to see how CBD oil could be used as an anti-cancer agent. Studies showed that CBD oil helped in preventing the growth of cancer cells in the body by blocking these cells from moving to different parts of the body. The example of Cash Hyde given above is a prime example of how CBD oil can be used to prevent cancer. This study shows that CBD helps in preventing the cancer cells from spreading across the body by killing these cells. CBD is non-toxic, and studies are being conducted to understand how the human body reacts on using CBD oil in comparison to the conventional treatments used for cancer.

In the medical community CBD oil has been known to affect the growth of tumors. Some studies have concluded that CBD oil can help to reduce the size of a tumor. There are antioxidants in CBD oil that help to lower the user's risk of cancer thanks to the anti-mutagenic properties.

Promotes Good Sleep

You can find a strong sedative quality in CBD oil that will help if you are having problems sleeping. When you inhale a small amount or place some on your chest, you will be able to get a good night's sleep.

Boost Immune System

A lot of cannabinoids have been proven to have positive effects on the immune system. CBD oil can help regulate an overactive immune system which will reduce the number of allergic reactions and also reduce the chance of procuring an autoimmune disease.

Chapter 2

Side Effects, Safety, and CBD Oil Legality

As with most treatments, there are potential side effects that you may or may not experience when using CBD oil. However, whenever CBD oil is used in moderate amounts, most people don't experience any side effects. None of the side effects of CBD oil have been known to be fatal or dangerous. In fact, there have been over 20,000 studies done in the last 15 years which have resulted in scientists concluding that cannabis, hemp, and cannabinoids are therapeutic.

Potential side effects:

- Dry mouth

- Lightheadedness

- Fatigue

- Impaired motor function

- Hypotension

If you are already having one of these conditions, you should be cautious when using CBD oil. Be sure to talk to your primary care physician before you use the oil because it could end up exacerbating your condition and if your doctor does not know, they are not going to know how to help if something goes wrong.

Keep the following precautions in mind when using CBD oil.

Blood Pressure

While CBD oil can help lower blood pressure and help protect your heart, (because of the calm feeling it promotes in the body) if you are already using a medication for hypertension and combine it with CBD oil, you may experience hypotension or low blood pressure.

Appropriate Use

Given that fatigue and lightheadedness is a side effect of CBD oil, especially if consumed in a large amount, you should be cautious when you are using heavy machinery, driving a vehicle, or something that requires concentration when it comes to your life and that of others. It is best that you do neither of these things until you know how CBD oil affects you. Whenever you use CBD oil, you may experience some feelings of sluggishness which can often be associated with the feeling of being high. This can end up causing motor functions to become impaired, but it is nothing to worry about because the effect is temporary and will pass in a few hours.

Weight Gain

Since CBD oil can be used to stimulate appetite or regulate it, you need to make sure to monitor your food intake, particularly if you are overweight.

Oil Quality

One of the most dangerous things about CBD oil use is the possibility of using low-quality oil or oil that has not been produced properly. Since there are thousands of small business that are trying to get into the medical marijuana industry, you need to ensure that you conduct thorough research on the brand and pay keen attention to customer reviews. If you are not careful, you could end up harming yourself due to a brand's negligence. We'll discuss this in detail in Chapter 9.

Pregnancy

It is not recommended to use CBD oil if you are pregnant. Some will say that it is great to use for depression, anxiety, and muscle aches. But, you are going to want to speak to your doctor before you try and use it on your own.

Is CBD Oil Safe?

As previously stated, there are some side effects when using CBD oil. However, it is safest when you do it under medical supervision. This is because there is no true dosage for CBD oil and you could end up taking too much. Not every person will experience the benefits of using CBD oil because everyone is different. It's also important to know that not every doctor is going to approve of the use of CBD oil.

Is CBD Oil Legal

Yes, CBD is legal throughout the entire world. In Canada, it is a controlled substance. But, there are a lot of misconceptions around CBD oil, especially when it comes to the chemical properties of the oil which are not fully understood yet. THC is a strictly controlled substance which causes CBD to be regulated. CBD is unrelated to the chemical chain that you find with THC. They share the same characteristics but are created from different paths.

Does CBD Oil Get You High?

No, CBD is a non-psychoactive, but you are going to feel more relaxed which most people associate with the feeling of being high. Since CBD oil does not have THC in it, you will not experience the paranoia that some people associate with cannabis. This is why CBD oil is legal.

Chapter 3

CBD Oil for Pain

Many people have questioned if CBD oil helps with the management of pain, and the research shows that it does. Various disorders like Diabetic Neuropathy, Multiple Sclerosis, and others attack the primary and the central nervous system which ends up leaving those who suffer from it in pain. Pain that's not easily controlled by common pain medication According to CBD oil clinical trials, the effects of CBD oil have been measured in how it helps with chronic pain management. It suggests that it can be used in an effort to increase the quality of life as well as allowing patients to rest without being in pain.

Some research even suggests that CBD oil is a good solution to those who may show sensitivity to other medications. At this point, government trials are being conducted to see how CBD oil will affect pain management and those who use it after a prolonged time.

CBD Dosage

Despite the fact that more and more states in the U.S. have legalized medical marijuana, a lot of doctors are hesitant to recommend cannabinoids since they are not 100% sure of the correct dosage to recommend. This is because medical schools rarely ever update their pharmacology courses.

You can find CBD oil in several different concentrations and forms. A flat dosage recommendation is not always the right dosage because everyone is different. A good rule of thumb is to start out small and increase gradually until the desired result is reached.

Different CBD oils will have different standards which lead to confusion amongst the consumers. A lot of them recommend too much while others do not recommend enough. Due to the lack of standard, a standard dosage would be 25 milligrams (mg) of CBD taken twice a day. It is also recommended that you increase the dosage everyone to four weeks by 25 milligrams until you experience relief. If you are experiencing worsening symptoms, then you will want to decrease it until you feel relief.

The Mayo clinic has done scientific research on cannabinoid dosages and how much should be taken depending on what you are suffering from. Here's what they had to say:

- Increasing appetite for cancer patients: 2.5 mg of THC by mouth with 1 mg of CBD for 6 weeks

- Chronic pain: 2.5 to 20mg by mouth for 25 days

- Epilepsy: 200-300 mg a day for 4 ½ months

- Movement problems tied to Huntington's: 10 mg per kilogram of CBD by mouth every day for 6 weeks

- Sleep disorders: 40-160 mg CBD by mouth

- Multiple sclerosis symptoms: THC-CBD mix 2.5 -120 mg every day by mouth for 2 to 15 weeks.

- Schizophrenia: 40-1,280 mg CBD by mouth for 4 weeks

- Glaucoma: 20-40 mg under your tongue. Anything greater than 40 mg may increase eye pressure

It is important to remember that the benefits of CBD oil always depend on the dosage administered.

CBD is usually taken orally in the form of tincture or drops and is placed under the tongue. Here are some general dosage guidelines that can be followed.

- General health: 2.5-15mg CBD to be taken orally, daily.
- For treating chronic pain: 2.5-20 mg CBD to be taken orally, daily.

- For treating sleep disorders: 40-160 mg CBD to be taken orally, daily.

Three Tips for Getting the Correct Dosage Of CBD

Well, how exactly will you be able to determine the right dosage? If you have never tried CBD, then there are a couple of things that you should be aware of. While CBD is used for treating seizures and epilepsy, pre-clinical evidence suggests that it can be made use of for treating anxiety, elevating mood, fighting pain, and reducing stress as well. However, the correct dosage of CBD would vary from one individual to another. A person who has epilepsy might need a higher dosage of CBD; while someone who is looking for a way to relax would need a small dosage of CBD. Keep these three tips in mind while you are trying to determine the correct dosage of CBD.

Start small:

When you are getting started with CBD, it is better if you start out with a small dosage. Everyone tends to react differently to different dosages. As with any new product, you will need to see how your body reacts to it. Depending on that reaction, you can take a call about increasing or decreasing the dosage. Elixinol has a low dosage of CBD, and this is a good way to get started. You can slowly work your way to your desired dosage. Get started with Elixinol 300 series for a small dosage.

Pay attention to the size:

The right dosage of CBD would vary from one person to another. As a general rule of thumb, a larger person might need a higher dosage of CBD than a smaller person. With CBD, you can amp up the dosage a few milligrams at a time for meeting your personal needs.

Always consult a medical professional:

If you have a medical condition, you should always refer to a healthcare professional before taking CBD. A doctor or a medical professional can tell you the way in which you are supposed to take it and the dosage so that you get the most out of it. So, always consult your doctor before getting started with this.

How to Use CBD Oil

CBD is usually taken orally in a concentrated paste, tincture form, or drops. To use the oil, hold it under your tongue so it can be absorbed in your mouth before you swallow. You must do this for the CBD to be broken down by the digestive system. There are other oral methods that you can take like mouth strips, edibles, and capsules. Some people prefer vape oil so that they can inhale the CBD and get instant relief. Other ways in which CBD oil can be used are to make lotions, balms, creams, and patches. There are many ways to use CBD oil that you may want to try. Figure out which one works for you.

Chapter 4

CBD Oil for Anxiety

Some of the early research has shown promising signs of how CBD oil can help relieve anxiety. It is believed that CBD oil works with brain receptors known as CB1 that are a part of the endocannabinoid system. These receptors are tiny proteins that are tied to your cells, and they take the chemical signals from various stimuli so that your cells know how to respond to what is going on inside of your body.

How CBD works with CB1 is not yet fully understood, but it is thought to modify serotonin signals. Serotonin is known as a feel-good chemical that works with your mental health. Whenever you have low serotonin levels, you may experience depression. And when you don't have enough serotonin in your body, you may also experience anxiety.

CBD is very effective when it comes to treating anxiety because of its effects on the brain. It is very important to remember that most of the known effects of CBD oil have been noted based on some preclinical studies and animal studies. There is a saying that goes, "Mice are not men"; therefore, it is important for us to remember that results from animal studies are not always true in the case of human beings. However, these results will lead us in the right direction.

5 - HT1A Agonist

5 – HT1A is a part of the serotonin system in the human body and is a type of serotonin receptor. This is an important element to consider since many medications used to treat depression and anxiety always target the serotonin system. This is why most of the medicines developed by drug companies are mostly serotonin reuptake inhibitors. These inhibitors help to prevent the brain from reabsorbing too much serotonin thereby increasing the serotonin that is available in the synaptic space. This helps the brain transmit

more serotonin signals throughout the body, which helps to boost a person's mood and reduce anxiety. However, the basis used to make this conclusion is complicated and not fully understood.

Similar to the Serotonin inhibitors, CBD helps the brain transmit more serotonin signals throughout the body. In an animal study conducted in Spain, researchers found that CBD improves and enhances the transmission of 5 – HT1A in the body and may show a faster impact when compared with the serotonin inhibitors that are available in pharmacies. The researchers concluded that CBD could be used to cure anxiety better than the drugs that are available in the market.

One of the most common treatments for low serotonin is to prescribe selective serotonin reuptake inhibitors otherwise known as SSRIs. Commonly prescribed medications that have SSRIs are Zoloft and Prozac. But, CBD is given to those who have trouble managing their anxiety. It is important for you to talk to your doctor before you change your treatment plan on your own, especially if you are thinking of using CBD oil with your SSRIs.

Hippocampal Neurogenesis

One of the most important parts of the brain is the hippocampus since it plays a critical role in a number of brain functions. This part plays a significant role in cognition and memory formation. Patients suffering from anxiety or depression have a smaller hippocampus. Treatment for depression is always successful when it is associated with generating new neurons (neurogenesis) in the hippocampus.

An animal study conducted on mice showed that the administration of CBD repeatedly helped to generate neurons in the hippocampus. If more research is being carried out on the differences between serotonin inhibitors and CBD oil in the future, this will open up new avenues that would help us understand anxiety and how to treat it effectively.

For general anxiety, the National Institute on Drug Abuse has stated that CBD has shown to lower stress level for animals. These subjects noticed lower behavioral signs of anxiety as well as lowered symptoms of anxiety such as an increased heart rate. Other studies show benefits to other forms of anxiety such as social anxiety, post-traumatic stress disorder, and even anxiety-induced insomnia.

In 2011, there was a human study on how CBD would affect someone who had social anxiety. The social anxiety subjects were given a placebo or 400 milligrams of CBD, and it showed that the patients that had CBD experienced lowered anxiety levels.

And a more recent study of CBD in psychiatric disorders, unfortunately, found inconclusive results. They could not see enough evidence to claim CBD as a realistic treatment for depression, but on a more positive note, it did show positive results for treating anxiety disorders. According to their review, an overwhelming majority of human tests need to undergo more reviews to better understand how it works, ideal dosages, and further side effects.

CBD has also been studied for other neurological disorders such as schizophrenia. In these studies, there have been reduced anxiety symptoms in both animals and humans when they used CBD. However, it is still shaky as to how it is going to make someone feel and what some of the side effects may be, especially if it is used with other anxiety medications. This is another reason why you should not self-diagnose yourself. Your medication may not be compatible with CBD and could cause a side effect no one knows about yet.

Studies on CBD Oil and Anxiety

A small double-blind study was conducted by Brazilian researchers using patients afflicted with social anxiety, as their subjects. Once the patients consumed CBD oil, they did show a significant decrease in the level of anxiety. The researchers then validated the subjective reports that the patients provided by performing scans of their brain. These scans showed blood flow patterns in the brain, which were consistent with the effect of anti-anxiety.

Another study conducted on patients suffering from Social Anxiety Disorder required them to perform a public speaking test that was simulated. Half the patients were administered with the CBD oil after which they were less anxious. The research findings were backed by the patients' blood pressure and heart rate. The researchers concluded that CBD reduced cognitive impairment, discomfort in speed performance and anxiety significantly. The other half, or the placebo group, were administered with regular treatment for anxiety. This half experienced higher discomfort, cognitive impairment, and anxiety.

Chapter 5

CBD Oil and Parkinson's Disease

Parkinson's is a progressive and chronic disorder that attacks the nervous system causing the brain's nerve cells to malfunction and eventually die. Parkinson's starts with a tremor that may never be noticed, but it gradually increases to where the body begins to experience stiffness and the slowing of their movements. Some neurons will produce dopamine to send out messages to the brain so the body can control its movement, but with Parkinson's these neurons die and the dopamine levels decrease as movement is affected.

Since the causes of Parkinson's are unknown, it is believed that genes and environmental triggers play a significant role. Some genetic mutations have been identified which is increasing the chance of figuring out what causes Parkinson's.

Parkinson's symptoms include the tremors, bradykinesia, rigidity, and even postural instability. Parkinson's doesn't just affect one part of the body, but all parts. This disease is typically accompanied by depression, problems sleeping, swallowing, cognitive problems, fatigue, and unrelenting pain. Eventually, the individual will suffer from psychosis which impairs how they think or react. In other words, they end up losing touch with reality, but psychosis does not occur in everyone.

At this point, there is no cure for Parkinson's but, there are treatments that are being used to improve the symptoms. Medications have been used to help with movement and tremors while surgery has been helped to regulate regions of the brain.

What about alternative treatment? Cannabis can slow the progression of Parkinson's by affecting the brain's neuroprotectant properties. The cannabinoids suppress excitotoxicity, oxidative injury, and glial activity. Along with helping stop the degeneration of dopamine neurons, cannabis has been shown to improve cells' mitochondrial function and the activity for cellular debris which further assists in encouraging healthy neurons.

Research has discovered that cannabinoid has assisted in the treatment of Parkinson's by preventing damage that is caused by free radicals and activating receptors that encourage the formation of new mitochondria. Cannabinoid can support the health of neural cells which researchers believe can be therapeutic to neurodegenerative disorders such as Parkinson's.

In another study, a patient that smoked cannabis saw major improvements in their symptoms while other studies have shown that it reduces tremors and bradykinesia.

While improvements in symptoms improve the quality of life for a Parkinson's patient, those who are given doses of CBD daily for a week experienced improved movement and did not have nearly as much pain if they had any at all. CBD has been ranked one of the most effective ways to treat Parkinson's over things such as vitamins, massage, and relaxation.

A recent study that was conducted by a team of Brazilian researchers showed that patients who have Parkinson's disease who were administered with CBD oil regularly showed an improved quality of life. Twenty-one such patients were administered with the oil through a gelatin capsule for a period of six weeks. Three different doses were administered – 300 mg per day, 75 mg per day and a placebo. Patients who were administered with the 300mg dosage showed the most improvement. However, it is important to note that the treatment did not affect the disease but affected the symptoms alone. But, some animal studies do suggest that CBD oil can be used to slow the progression of the disease and certain other neurodegenerative diseases.

It is safe to say that CBD oil can help to alleviate a range of health conditions, deficiencies, and problems. There is a lot more research that would need to be conducted to understand the effects of CBD on the human body in detail.

Study on CBD Oil and Parkinson's Disease

The Department of Neurology, Beilinson Hospital and the Sackler Faculty of Medicine from Tel Aviv University conducted a study to identify and understand the effects of CBD oil on Parkinson's disease.

CBD Oil has been used as a therapeutic agent for a number of medical conditions, and these methods have been documented well. However, clinical trials held where patients who have Parkinson's disease were administered with CBD oil have yielded conflicting results. This study aimed to assess the effect of CBD oil on the non-motor and motor symptoms of Parkinson's disease.

Twenty-two patients who were attending the motor disorder clinic of a medical center between the years 2011 and 2012 were all evaluated under standard conditions and also evaluated after using inhaling the diffused CBD oil for thirty minutes. They were all assessed using the following:

- Present Pain Intensity Scale

- Visual Analog Scale

- Unified Parkinson Disease Rating Scale

- Short – Form McGill Pain Questionnaire

- Medical Cannabis Survey

- National Drug and Alcohol Research questionnaire

After the consumption of CBD oil, the mean total score on the motor Unified Parkinson Disease Rating Scale improved from 33.1 under standard conditions to 23.2. There was also an improvement in the pain scores and also the sleep of the patient.

No significant side effects were observed. Larger studies are needed to verify the results obtained.

Chapter 6

CBD Oil for ADD and ADHD

ADD, and ADHD can be traced back to a chemical imbalance in the brain.

These conditions make it difficult to complete a task. When asked to complete a task, they can easily become frustrated. It is easy for people to encourage them to change their behavior simply, but it's not that simple.

Some people outgrow ADD and ADHD, but there is still around 4.4% of adults suffer from this disease. ADD, and ADHD patients can become chronically bored, impulsive, and even have poor organizational skills. These symptoms put a strain on relationships and cause people to fall behind in their work tasks as well as increasing their risk for mental disorders.

What's the cause? Prominent level of cortisol and low levels of dopamine can be what causes someone to suffer from ADD and ADHD symptoms. CBD controls levels of cortisol while increasing the levels of dopamine which in effect reduce the symptoms of ADD and ADHD.

While it is controversial to give small children CBD oil, if you truly want to get ahead of the symptoms that come with ADD and ADHD then it is best to attempt to give them the oil while they are young. CBD oil can still be used in patients who are older to improve their ability to finish tasks and put their ADD or ADHD behind them.

Studies on CBD Oil and ADD and ADHD

ADHD and ADD are the most common disorders in children, but these can persist even in adult years. The chronic conditions are often not curable although treatment can be sought for the same. Unfortunately for some patients, the usual treatment does not prove to be effective. So how can they treat themselves? Research says that CBD oil is the next best contender.

In the year 2013, a study that was published in the Journal of Substance Use and Misuse found that most people, to handle hyperactivity and their impulsive nature (two most common components of ADD and ADHD), were self-medicating.

The study surveyed about 280 users of CBD oil, and the finding was that most people experienced stronger symptoms of ADD and ADHD when they were not on self-medication. This finding led to studying and understanding the link that exists between CBD and the endocannabinoid system in the human body.

After the study that was conducted in 2013, German researchers sought to examine the relationship between ADD and CBD closely. They used a sample of 30 patients who were resisting traditional treatments between 2013 and 2014. They published their findings in the year 2015.

There were 2 female patients and 28 male patients (since ADD and ADHD are more common in men) between the ages of 21 and 51 with the mean age being between 30 years. In the case of each patient, it was found that there was a lot of improvement in sleep. Although the study was small, the researchers were confident that CBD oil could be used to treat patients who have ADD and ADHD, especially patients who were resisting traditional treatment.

Chapter 7

CBD Oil and Alzheimer's

Alzheimer's is one of the most common forms of dementia that currently affects over 4.5 million people, and studies have shown cannabis can limit the progression of the disease. Alzheimer's is progressive dementia that takes away a person's memory, ability to think, and behavior. The brain cells degenerate to the point that they die and cause memory decline as well as a decline of social and intellectual skills. As brain cells die, the brain shrinks along with it over time.

Alzheimer's begins with, forgetfulness or mild confusion. It then progresses, and the rate that it advances depends on the person. Their memory gets worse over time which causes them to repeat what they have said, like asking the same question multiple times, misplace things, or forget a family member's name. They lose their sense of day and can't find the proper word to express what they are trying to say. Additionally, they can't fully understand or experience depression, mood swings, irritability, or other mental disorders.

At the moment, there is no cure for this disease, and medications provide a temporary improvement in the symptoms. The Mayo clinic believes Alzheimer's is caused from environmental, lifestyle and genetic factors. Age seems to also play a role in those who have Alzheimer's. Patients are typically sixty-five and older.

THC has been shown to lower amyloid beta levels while enhancing mitochondrial functions which cause researchers to believe that THC could be a potential therapeutic treatment option for Alzheimer's through multiple functions and pathways.

Someone with Alzheimer's will experience an over-activation of microglia which causes brain tangles. But, CBD has shown that it can modulate microglial functions as well as control inflammation in the brain. CBD can improve the survival rate of cells through the properties that CBD holds to help with inflammation and the buildup to toxicity. Cannabinoids work at providing a multi-facet approach when it comes to treating Alzheimer's because it promotes a healthy brain.

It is not conclusive that CBD can stop Alzheimer's permanently, but it can slow down the progression of the disease. This is one of the best treatments that have been found to help with Alzheimer's patients.

Study on CBD Oil and Alzheimer's disease

Alzheimer's disease is often caused due to the formation of certain compounds called beta-amyloid plaques in the brain. Researchers have managed to prove that medical marijuana can be used to fight the formation of the plaque in the brain. However, they were not able to show that medical marijuana can be used to treat Alzheimer's.

A research team at Radboud University Medical Center in Netherlands had recently investigated the effects of medical marijuana on Alzheimer's and its symptoms including anxiety, depression, aggression, hallucinations, and insomnia. They did not see a significant statistical difference when medical marijuana was used to treat the symptoms associated with Alzheimer's.

The research team divided the fifty participants into two groups. One group was administered with a pill that had 1.5 mg of medical marijuana, and the other group was administered with a placebo pill three times a day. The behavioral symptoms of the two groups were compared for three weeks, and it was found that there was a slight difference between the behaviors of the members of the two groups.

Another study that was published in The Journal of Alzheimer's Disease has concluded that an extract of cannabis with a higher concentration of CBD can help to relieve the symptoms associated with Alzheimer's

A group of researchers from the Sackler Faculty of Medicine at the Tel Aviv University, the Abarbanel Mental Health Center and the Department of Psychology at Barilan University conducted a study, which was the first clinical study that observed the effect of cannabis on patients who have Alzheimer's.

The study found the effects of CBD on a group of 11 people who have Alzheimer's for four weeks. Ten of the participants survived the trial. Although the sample was too small, the researchers concluded that adding CBD oil to the patients' therapy has promising results and is safe.

Chapter 8

Fibromyalgia and CBD

Fibromyalgia is a musculoskeletal pain that affects around five million people. There have been multiple studies done to show that CBD can lower the pain levels and increase the quality of sleep in the individuals who have fibromyalgia.

This disorder is typically described as a widespread pain and fatigue that targets women primarily. This disorder can cause someone to have difficulty performing daily tasks and sleep disruption. Fibromyalgia is severe because the brain is taking the body's pain signals and amplifying them. Since these pain signals are amplified, the patient suffering from fibromyalgia will experience times where they can't get out of bed to do anything. To make matters worse, laying down can sometimes trigger painful symptoms. Those who suffer from fibromyalgia also have memory problems along with other cognitive issues, stiffness in the morning, headaches, numbness and tingling, painful menstrual periods, sensitivity to temperature, restless leg syndrome, depression, and irritable bowel syndrome.

The cause of fibromyalgia is unknown, but the National Institute of Arthritis and Musculoskeletal and Skin Diseases says people who suffer from this disease tie it to being physically or emotionally stressed or a traumatic event. Things such as repetitive illnesses or injuries are associated with fibromyalgia. Others have claimed that their disorder came out of the blue. Unfortunately, there has been no cure found for fibromyalgia, but those that are receiving treatment have focused pain management.

All cannabinoids have analgesic and sleep-promoting effects that allow patients to manage their symptoms daily. Along with improving sleep, cannabinoids help with the stiffness that patients feel in their joints and the anxiety they feel from not being able to complete all their tasks.

Fibromyalgia patients that have been treated with CBD have been watched over a seven-month period, and they showed significant improvements in their pain levels as well as reducing how many opioids they were taking. A four-week study showed that the patients that were given CBD could get through their day easier while those who received the placebo did not have any improvements. In yet another study, fibromyalgia patients who received CBD were not only experiencing less pain and sleeping better, but they were able to relax better than before.

Study on CBD Oil and Fibromyalgia

The Human Pharmacology and Neurosciences Unit Institut de Recerca Hospital del Mar-IMIM, Parc de Salut Mar, Barcelona, Spain conducted a study on the effects of CBD oil on patients suffering from Fibromyalgia.

The purpose of their study was to explain the benefits associated with using certain display of cannabis on patients with fibromyalgia. The researchers also compared the quality of life of the patients who were administered the cannabis with the patients who used traditional medicine. They measured the perceived benefits of using CBD oil on patients with a range of symptoms using the standard visual analogue scale (VAS). The information on how much cannabis was being administered to patients was recorded using a questionnaire. CBD oil users and non-users completed the Fibromyalgia Impact Questionnaire (FIQ), the Pittsburgh Sleep Quality Index (PSQI) and the Short Form 36 Health Survey (SF-36).

There was a total of fifty-six patients – twenty-eight of them were administered with CBD oil while the other twenty-eight were using traditional medicine. The demographics of the groups were the same. CBD users were administered with the drug in different forms – smoking, oral and combined. The dosage and the frequency of the drug were also different for each patient. After using CBD for two hours, the VAS score for the patients was statistically lower which implied that there was a reduction in the pain and stiffness that the patients felt. The patients were more relaxed and were more active.

The use of cannabis is linked with beneficial results on a few FM symptoms. Advanced studies on the efficiency of cannabinoids in people suffering from FM as well as cannabinoid structure contribution in the pathophysiology of FM are warranted.

Chapter 9

Buying CBD Oil

Where to Buy CBD Oil

A lot of people want to buy CBD oil online because they think they must live in a state that has legalized medical marijuana to purchase CBD oil legally. But, this is not true because CBD oil is produced from industrial hemp. When you are looking to buy CBD oil, online or offline, remember that not all CBD products are the same. CBD oil is legal if it is produced from industrial hemp. If it is produced from medical marijuana, it will still be subject to the laws and regulations of the respective state.

The main difference between CBD oil that is produced from hemp is, and CBD oil produced from marijuana is it's not going to have any THC. That also makes it safe to consume which means that it is legal in the United States and at least forty countries around the world.

Make sure that you do proper research when it comes to which experts to trust. People who claim that they are experts on marijuana are a dime a dozen, especially online. This doesn't mean that real experts aren't out there; however, because medical marijuana gets attention true experts have emerged. A website known as healthy hemp oil (www.healthyhempoil.com) focuses on cannabidiol products, and they strive to make sure they are giving their customer the healthiest and most trusted oil products.

Whenever you are thinking about trying a new type of CBD oil, it is important to check consumer reviews for your due diligence. You never know what additional ingredients could end up in products purchased online and sticking with the highest quality and well-known products will keep you in the clear.

Best Rated CBD Oil

You can find the following oils at healthyhempoil.com.

Herbal Renewals: Blue Label High CBD Hemp Oil (150 mg, 450 mg, and 1500 mg)

This is one of the purest versions of CBD oil available on the market which means that there are no fillers or flavors added. This product is as close to Rick Simpson oil (we'll discuss this oil in chapter 14) and Real Scientific Hemp Oil that you can get.

Herbal Renewals: CBD Oil Herbal Spray (100 – 500 mg)

Tinctures are one of the most popular forms of CBD oil, so there are a lot of options for you to pick from. Tinctures are usually better than other CBD forms due to the fact it uses high-quality ingredients, it is effective, and it is easy to use. This spray makes use of CBD oil easy by allowing you to spray it under your tongue. Once sprayed, allow it to dissolve. You'll feel the effects afterward. This CBD spray comes in peppermint, vanilla, and it can come as unflavored as well.

Tasty Hemp Oil: Tasty Vape Oil (250 mg)

Vape oils are usually known for being low quality and use synthetic ingredients, but this vape oil is not like that. With Tasty Hemp Oil, you can pick from seven assorted flavors all of which are some sort of fruit flavor to give you that extra burst when you are using it.

Herbal Renewals: CBD Oil Herbal Spray (100 – 500 mg)

If you are new to using CBD oil, then start with this product because it is easy to use and you'll get the best bang for your buck.

There are plenty of other CBD products out there, but these are some of the best available. These use pure ingredients and are not harmful.

Research Your Potential CBD Oil Products

How do you know if you're looking at an inferior product? Let's take these instructions found on a CBD product for example:

With this spray, you will get 80 servings (1.25 mg each) of premium quality all natural and extra strong CBD oil. Simply spray twice on your tongue and get an instant taste of CBD goodness with no hassle and a tasty kick.

After researching this company's products (Plus CBD Oil), you'll find that their CBD comes from Austria farms that have special cultivators to grow hemp plants without any chemicals as well as making the plants non-GMO. Once they have been planted and are growing, a third party comes in and tests the plants to ensure that the process is done correctly. Once harvested, it will be manufactured in California. It's always good to do a background check on how a company's products are made.

It's also good to notice the milligrams in product's labels. Usually, one bottle has at least 100 milligrams of CBD and is sold for around $47. However, when you look at the higher-priced products, they are cheaper per milligram of CBD than the smaller more affordable bottles.

Now, look at the ingredients of this CBD bottle:

Natural flavoring, hemp oil (seed and stalk), potassium sorbate, cannabidiol (CBD), lecithin, stevia extract, emulsifier (Sorbian monooleate), kosher vegetable glycerin, water.

The biggest issue here is that sorbates are primarily used as a food preservative. A food preservative! While we are constantly placing sorbate in our body because of our food, why would we want to place it in our bodies when it comes to oil that is supposed to help overcome health issues?

Go to Kannaway website (kannaway.com) and research what they're all about for practice. Their ingredients don't have any preservatives, and their flavors are true fruit extracts. Not only that, but their formula adds value and enhances the effects that you feel from CBD oil.

Red flags to look out for are synthetic chemicals in your CBD oil because of its ties to DNA toxins. Pay attention to labels when you're shopping online, so you are not buying knock-off oil or placing harmful chemicals in your body with a product that is supposed to be natural and helpful.

Chapter 10

Growing Cannabis Plants and Making CBD Oil

Step by Step Growing Process

1. Select where you're going to grow your plant(s). If you're using a grow room, then make sure that your room is set up for the number of plants that you plan on growing. Ensure that everything is set up (from the lights to the fans to the water drainage). If you're growing outside, ensure that your soil has been tilled and that there are no rocks or weeds that could end up killing your plants in the long run.

2. Seeds may just seem like seeds, but different seeds yield different strains. So, we must select our seeds according to the strains we want. Sativa, hybrids, or Indica strains are just some of the few that you can choose from, but make sure that you

get feminized seeds. You can simply find these through some online searching.

3. Next, you're going to need to get a container. Many different containers will work. However, I suggest you start out with a fabric growing pot to ensure that your roots get the oxygen.

4. The soil you use is also extremely important to your long-term success. If you aren't sure what type of soil is best suited to your needs and climate, don't be afraid to ask a professional gardener or do some online research. Once you have selected your perfect soil, fill your pot with soil to grow your plants. Different seeds will have different growing instructions. Thus, be mindful of this when you start the growing process. While you fill the pot, don't pack your dirt down. The soil is best left fluffy. This is to ensure that your roots can take proper hold and your plant receives its proper nutrients.

5. At this point, your pot will be ready for your seeds. Place your seeds 1-1.5 inches into the soil. It

won't be too deep that water won't get to it, but it won't be so shallow that the roots won't be able to take hold. Water your seeds after you have planted them.

It is also important that you don't let the soil dry out while you're going through the sprouting phase but at the same time don't overwater it. Just ensure that the soil stays moist daily.

6. Give it light. By keeping an eye on your plant, you'll notice that baby leaves will begin to sprout. When you see leaves, begin to give your plants proper lighting. Cannabis needs a lot of light so ensure that you've gotten the right light bulbs for the job. LED lights are widely used when you're growing. However, you can also use a 600-watt sodium lamp to ensure your plants are getting the light they need. During the growing process, make sure to give your plants a steady eighteen hours of light each day.

7. When you're watering your plants, wait until the top inch of soil has become dry more water –

do this to avoid overwatering. Plant food can be used during the growing process to ensure that your plant is getting its needed nutrients in case your soil isn't doing the job. Like soil, the nutrients you use on your plants can make the difference between serious yields and tiny, malnourished buds.

8. You'll also need to initiate the flowering process. The way to do this is to slowly take away the amount of light that your plant is receiving to initiate the changing in seasons that wild weed experiences. To do this, you can scale the light back to about twelve hours a day before placing it in pure darkness for the other twelve hours a day. This will imitate the long summer days turning into the darker days allowing your plants to flower.

How to Make CBD Oil

You can make cannabis oil by separating the resin that you extract from the flower of the plant. Cannabis oil is extremely popular because of how simple it is to make. It's recommended to at least get an ounce of cannabis to get the best results for your oil.

To start, you should be working in an environment that is opened so that fumes can escape or be blown away from your workspace to ensure you don't breathe in harmful fumes – lab vents are best. Also, make sure that you have a fire extinguisher on hand (just in case) because your workspace will be flammable. If there is propane or other flammable objects near your workspace, remove them. Also, stick to electrical tools if possible to be safe.

You will have to use a gallon of high proof alcohol. The higher the proof, the more potent your oil will end up being when all the solvents are burned off. Do not use rubbing alcohol because there are other properties found in rubbing alcohol that can harm you if you make your oil with it.

Other tools you'll need are a mixing bowl, spatula, strainer, a wooden spoon, a rice cooker or double boiler, and syringes, so you don't waste any of your oil when you are putting it in the containers for storage.

A final precaution is proper safety gear to protect yourself from chemicals that you can get exposed to. Get ready safety glasses, gloves, oven mitts, hot pads, and a mask. The mask is going to prevent the fumes from getting into your lungs.

Once you have gathered everything, have it close by. Then take your cannabis and soak it in the high proof alcohol solvent. The alcohol needs to completely cover your marijuana in the mixing bowl you are using. If you do not know how much alcohol to use, have at least an inch of solvent above your cannabis that should be sitting in the bottom of the bowl under the alcohol.

With your spoon mix the solvent into the cannabis. Mash the cannabis up to get the best results. By doing this, you are letting the solvent completely saturate the bud not just on the outside, but on the inside as well. Stir for about three minutes to ensure that all the THC is taken out of the bud.

Take another bowl and place it in the strainer and strain the solvent into the bowl. The liquid that you see will be a dark green color. Now, use your hands or spoon and get as much of the alcohol out of the bud as you can. We want as much of the THC into the liquid bowl.

This is only the first time that you'll strain the cannabis. You'll have around seventy to eighty percent of the resin that the bud produced. Take the cannabis and put it back in the bowl and repeat the process again. After you complete the stirring process, you will strain it once more to get a green liquid like you did the first time.

Once you have gotten all the resin from the cannabis, you will be at the point where you can burn the solvent off the oil so that it can be used. To do this, place some water into the double boiler before putting your liquid pan on top of it. Ensure that the boiler is on high heat and it boils. Whenever it starts to boil, the solvent is going to burn off. You do not want it to boil too long, or you risk losing resin. The ideal time will be about twenty-five seconds before you move to scraping the sides of the pan so that it does not stick.

If the liquid is still runny when the boiling process stops, turn the boiler on low heat and allow it to bubble. Once it has bubbled, turn the heat off. The liquid should resemble a syrup in the pan. If this is what you have, and then have successfully boiled off all the high proof alcohol.

Allow the oil to cool before you attempt to move on to the next step. While the oil is cooling, expect it to thicken.

You'll most likely not use all the oil at once so store it once it has completely cooled down. Store it in one of the oral syringes and use it as needed. Another storage alternative is to put it in a glass jar that is completely sealed. Once you have it in the storage container of your choice, place it in a cool and shaded area.

How to Extract CBD?

There are different ways to extract CBD from hemp plants. The most common methods used have been described in this section.

CO_2 Method

The name speaks for itself – CO_2 is used in the extraction process. CO_2, which is at low temperature and under high pressure, is passed through the plant. This would lead to the extraction of the chemical in its purest form. This is considered the best process since CBD is extracted in its pure form along with the removal of the other cannabinoids and chemical compounds like chlorophyll. CBD extracted through this process has the best taste. The downside to this process is that it is an expensive process.

Ethanol Method

Ethanol is a high grain alcohol, and it is administered to the plant in the same way as CO_2 is administered to the plant. A disadvantage of this process is that it could destroy some of the acids that are found in the plant.

Oil Method

This method has been gaining immense popularity in the recent years. The process involves the extraction of the chemical using certain carrier oils, like olive oil, almond oil, and coconut oil. The carrier oil that is used most often is olive oil since it has certain properties that would enhance the properties of the CBD extracted. It is for this reason that this process is being used more often. The chemical that is extracted from this process is also free of any residue.

Chapter 11

Cancer, CBD and Hemp Oils

Cancer is defined as a cell that is in the human body that has unchecked growth which endangers the host when it spreads. With the growth comes inflammation and compression of tissue and organs nearby which causes painful symptoms.

The most common cancer treatment is chemotherapy and radiation, but both cause the breakdown of healthy tissue as well as unnecessary inflammation. The biggest thing that people are going through cancer treatments experience is the pain, nausea, and a loss of appetite.

Clinical trials suggest that cannabinoids can be used so the patient can regain their appetite and avoid the pain that cancer causes. Recent studies have shown CBD oil and cancer treatments can have a synergistic effect, therefore, causing the treatment to work better than it would have before.

Some main benefits that CBD oil provides when it comes to cancer are:

- Antiviral activity

- Anti-inflammatory activity

- The prevention of growth in the blood vessels that will supply tumors.

- Harmful cell growth blocked

Hemp Oil

There's a special type of hemp oil called Rick Simpson Oil we'll go over in chapter 14 coming up soon. For now, let's get familiar with hemp oil.

Some people think that hemp oil is a miracle substance that can cure multiple diseases. And that people are not allowed to use it because the big pharmaceutical companies don't want to lose money on a cure that everyone can get their hands on.

At Harvard University study showed the THC in marijuana could cut tumor growth down in lung cancer while also reducing the ability for cancer to spread. One of the first things that the experiment showed was that THC could activate the receptors that were naturally produced by the body to fight off lung cancer. In fact, a British pilot study showed that whenever doses of THC were injected into mice that had been given the human lung cancer cells, the tumors shrunk and even killed the cells.

Therefore, both CBD and hemp oil can help reduce the inflammation and shrink tumors found in cancer patients. CBD oil and cancer treatments such as chemo and radiation have given patients and easier experience in getting over their cancer by reducing the pain symptoms they experience. They can also eat without worrying about not being able to keep the food down.

While each medical doctor does not always approve CBD and hemp oil, it has been studied and shows improve the treatment of cancer. As the patient, you can choose how you treat your cancer, and if you want to use CBD or hemp oil, find a doctor that has experience with these oils so that you are not self-treating and potentially harming yourself.

Studies on CBD Oil and Cancer

A number of studies are being carried out in trying to understand how CBD oil could be used to treat cancer. Many studies show that CBD oil can be used to kill cancer cells in the body or prevent them from moving to different parts of the body.

Breast cancer is a disease that is the second most common cause of death in women. Studies that were published the National Cancer Institute in the US claimed that CBD oil could be used to kill breast cancer cells that are found in the body. There are two other benefits one gains from using CBD oil after undergoing chemo. The first benefit is the increase in appetite. Chemo often reduces a patient's appetite, and CBD oil can be used to increase it. The second benefit is very obvious – it helps to alleviate the pain that cancer patients feel after undergoing multiple rounds of chemo.

Recent studies show that CBD oil and a number of other cannabinoids found in cannabis help to slow down the growth of cancer cells in the body. CBD oil was used on cancer cells that were grown in lab dishes to see how cancer cells react to CBD oil. Some studies were also conducted on animals to see how CBD oil could effectively help to slow down the growth of cannabinoids and help to reduce the migration of certain cancer cells across the body.

Early clinical trials conducted on human beings have concluded that CBD oil certainly has an effect on cancer cells and also helps to slow the growth of them. However, these studies do not show that CBD oil can be used to cure cancer. There are a number of other studies that have been planned to understand the extent to which CBD oil can be used to treat cancer.

Two drugs have been approved by the FDA to be used in the US to help cancer patients:

- Dronabinol: This is a gelatin capsule that contains THC which has been approved by the FDA to help treat vomiting and nausea that is caused due to chemotherapy. It also helps to increase the patient's appetite thereby increasing their weight.

- Nabilone: This is a synthetic cannabinoid and acts like the THC and CBD. This is taken orally to treat vomiting and nausea that is caused by chemotherapy. This drug is used only when other drugs fail to work. This drug has still not been approved but is being tests in a number of clinical trials to see how it helps cancer patients.

The American Cancer Society has stated that more research will need to be conducted on the use of CBD and other cannabinoids for cancer patients. It also recognizes that better therapies would need to be identified to reduce the pain and other side effects that cancer patients go through on account of the treatment they are subjected to.

Chapter 12

Hemp Oil

Hemp oil is used similarly to CBD oil. It helps with health issues that people experience such as depression and anxiety. Not only that, but it's used topically to help with skin issues.

Here's a taste of how hemp oil can help.

- Eczema: A study found that those who used hemp seed oil had their eczema vanish because of the strong anti-inflammatory properties that are in the oil.

- Multiple Sclerosis: While this is a dangerous and rare condition, the oil extract along with Evening Primrose Oil has been able to improve an MS patient's health.

- Inflammation: The omega and fatty acids found in hemp oil lower the systemic inflammation that people suffer from due to conditions such as arthritis.

- Acne: Whenever used topically; it prevents breakouts unlike some of the leading acne products found in a store.

Other uses for hemp oil are:

- It can be used as moisturizing oil since it is natural. After you bathe, you can massage your body with it to not only nourish your skin but to improve your blood circulation.

- It is a safe replacement for petroleum jelly. It is not toxic and doesn't to harm the environment.

The Benefits of Hemp Oil

Hemp oil has a lot of different benefits, and it provides amino acids to the body when used in its rawest forms.

Skin

Hemp oil has a lot of fatty acids that are great for your skin. These acids nourish and moisturize your skin when it is used in the proper manner and right amount. Some skin products such as face and body creams use hemp oil as their number one ingredient. Hemp seed oil is herbal, and there little to no side effects. When you get a massage with only hemp oil, you'll give your skin the vitamins and essential fatty acids it needs to keep your skin young and healthy. If you use hemp oil regularly, you may notice an anti-aging benefit as well. It also works to prevent conditions such as dry skin, psoriasis, acne, and eczema.

Hair

A lot of non-commercial herbal hair products use hemp oil. Hemp oil can increase blood circulation to your head and brain. When you wash your hair with hemp oil, you may realize that your hair thickens and you are experiencing less to no dandruff. Scalp infections and hair loss are also reduced.

Alpha Linolenic Acid

Hemp oil has been found to contain a lot of alpha-linolenic acid, and this acid is an omega 3 acid that assists vital organs. You can find this same acid in fish oil, and it also helps prevent heart disease.

Side Effects

Hemp oil may be used in the treatment of small health ailments and used as a dietary supplement to promote good health. Although the side effects of using hemp oil are slim, below are some precautions. Make sure to speak to your medical provider about using hemp oil and how it can potentially affect you.

Peroxides

Do not use hemp oil for frying food. You should only use it when you are preparing cold and warm dishes that are not going to get heated higher than

121 °F. High heat breaks down the polyunsaturated fats that result in peroxide production. You should never use it as a substitute for frying oils. Keep it in the fridge or freezer after you open the bottle.

Digestive Symptoms

There have been mentions that using hemp oil can soften your stools which end up causing abdominal cramping and diarrhea. Excessive diarrhea leads to weight loss or experiencing malabsorption. There must be further research to make sure that these claims are real. But, it is recommended that if you suffer from digestive disorders or irregular bowel movements, you should not use hemp oil or hemp oil supplements. As stated previously, please check with your medical provider before trying any new supplement.

THC

Users have claimed that hemp oil can cause the same feelings that you get from smoking marijuana. Make sure to be in a safe and calm environment when using hemp oil.

Blood

Hemp oil can affect the anticoagulant properties that are found in platelets in the blood which will halt or stall the production of these platelets. This can cause patients to experience complications if they are being treated for any blood clotting deficiencies or cardiac medical conditions.

CBD Oil Facts

Before you officially decide to use CBD oil and hemp oil, it's good to understand the facts about CBD and hemp.

Here are 3 CBD oil facts.

1. CBD is the key ingredient in cannabis. It is just one of the sixty compounds that you find in a cannabis plant. Through selective breeding, those who grow cannabis can create various levels of

CBD and THC in plants. These strains are rare but are slowly beginning to become more popular.

2. CBD is a non-psychoactive. You are not going to get high off CBD. Therefore, CBD is a poor choice for those who use cannabis recreationally, but it gives other advantages to the progressive field of medicine since it does not have many side effects. CBD is not psychoactive because it doesn't act on the same pathway that THC uses.

3. There are a lot of medical benefits from using CBD oil. Even though it uses a different pathway than THC, there are similar medical benefits from both.

Here are some of the medical properties and effects that you get from CBD:

- Antiemetic – reduces vomiting and nausea.
- Anxiolytic and antidepressant – works to fight anxiety and depression disorders.

- Anticonvulsant – reduces and even stops seizure activity.

- Anti - tumoral and anti-cancer – fights tumors and cancer cells.

- Antipsychotic – combats multiple psychosis disorders that people suffer from.

- Antioxidant – works to combat neurodegenerative disorders.

- Anti-inflammatory – lowers inflammatory disorders.

Most of these results come from animal studies rather than humans because there have not been many scientific studies carried out on human patients. However, there are lots of CBD testimonials. A pharmaceutical company in the United Kingdom developed a pharmaceutical version of CBD which is now funding trials for epilepsy and schizophrenia – so progress is being made.

Hemp Oil Facts

1.   The seeds produce the best hemp oil even though you can use the whole plant to make oil. Oil that has been cold pressed will have a rich and nutty flavor as well as a green tint. Once it has been refined, hemp oil will be colorless and almost flavorless.

2.   A classic way to use hemp oil is soaps. There are many other health and skincare products that you'll find contain hemp oil in them because of the amino acids, omega 3s, and vitamins found hemp oil.

3.   Hemp that is not refined will not have a long shelf life. The oil will quickly become rancid unless placed in a dark container in an environment like a refrigerator. Those who use unrefined hemp will purchase it in insignificant amounts so that it does not become rancid. Hemp oil is not suitable for cooking since it has a low smoke point. Refined hemp will have a longer shelf life although some of

the benefits will be removed since it has been refined.

4. Being that hemp is such a controversial crop in some parts of the world, hemp has become banned even though products that are made from hemp are allowed. In other parts of the world, only industrial hemp is allowed; some have been allowed to grow hemp without bans. In these areas, it is easier to regulate the growth of the plant instead of banning it all together which will cause people to grow it behind the government's back. Wild hemp is not too uncommon in some parts of the world which make it difficult to enforce a ban on hemp crops.

Hemp Oil and Nutrition

As mentioned earlier, hemp oil is extracted from the hemp plant. The oil contains around 80% polyunsaturated fatty acids which are considered to be good for the human body and 10% of the fatty acids that our body does not need. Hemp oil is one of the most unsaturated oils that are extracted from various plants. Unsaturated fatty acids are very important for the human body, sometimes more important when compared with vitamins, but our body is incapable of producing them. These fatty acids would need to be obtained from external sources and are extremely important for us to exist. These fatty acids are important for our energy levels.

Hemp oil is considered by most people to be the most balanced oil that is obtained in nature. This oil has the perfect ratio of Omega six and Omega three fatty acids. These two fatty acids are extremely essential for the human body. Hemp oil also contains certain other polyunsaturated fatty acids like stearidonic acid, oleic acid, and gamma-linolenic acid (GLA). These characteristics are what make hemp oil the most balanced oil.

Human beings can procure a number of diseases because of the deficiency of fatty acids in the body. There are a few disorders that one could procure if there are imbalances of these acids in the human body. Most often, diseases in the human body arise due to the lack of omega six and omega three or their derivatives. These fatty acids are not only sources of energy, but also important for good skin. These fats also help to enhance the stamina of the immune system. However, these fatty acids could either be produced in minimal amounts due to some defects in the enzyme system.

To treat any of these disorders, doctors usually prescribe drugs or dietary supplements that could often have side effects. However, it is better to use hemp oil since this oil has a good amount of these fatty acids. It would be better to use hemp oil instead of the drugs often prescribed since hemp oil does not have too many side effects.

In addition to the fatty acids, hemp oil also contains a number of antioxidants like phospholipids, carotene, Vitamin E, and phytosterols. Hemp oil also contains a number of minerals like magnesium, calcium, sulfur, potassium, phosphorous and small amounts of iron and zinc.

Chapter 13

The Difference between Hemp, Cannabis, and More

The difference between cannabis and hemp is in use. Both marijuana and hemp come from the same plant. However, the term hemp refers to the commercial and industrial use of the cannabis stalk and seeds for various objects. The term marijuana refers to the medical and recreational use of the cannabis flower.

Hemp typically has 0.3 to 1.5 percent THC while marijuana has as much as 30 percent more. Hemp fiber is long, strong, and more durable than all other natural fibers. Hemp cultivation doesn't require any chemicals such as herbicides or pesticides. It is grown in rotation with other crops like corn.

Hemp farming is completely sustainable. Most hemp farms produce about four times as much fiber as an acre of a pine tree would. Hemp can produce tree-free paper that can be recycled and reused up to seven times since hemp is easy to grow and will condition the soil that it grows in. The seeds and seed oil for hemp are full of protein and amino acids. Hemp is one of the most ideological sources for biomass fuels, and hemp ethanol burns fairly clean.

Industrial hemp is a type of cannabis that is used in the United States. Hemp has been associated with marijuana since the 1930's and where it became a versatile crop that was doomed to obscurity for decades. Hemp, while in the same species as marijuana is vitally different than cannabis. Hemp has a low THC level as discussed earlier. If you want to get the same psychoactive effect that you get from smoking marijuana, you will have to smoke up to twelve hemp cigarettes in an abbreviated period of time. Hemp has a lower THC content because THC forms in resin glands on the flowers of a female cannabis plant. Furthermore, hemp has a higher content of the chemical cannabidiol.

Cannabis, visually, has lower fiber content whereas hemp has strong fibers. This fiber has a wealth of everyday uses. The fibers from the marijuana plant have a low tensile strength and will shred faster, therefore, making it a poor fibrous plant when you compare it to hemp.

Industrial hemp is grown differently than cannabis. Hemp is usually grown vertically up instead of out because you are not focusing on producing buds, but rather on the length of the stalk, this causes hemp to be similar to bamboo. The stalk contains fiber and has a hard and woody core that is used in a variety of projects. Usually, marijuana plants grow to a height of five feet while hemp is going to grow to fifteen feet before harvested. The hemp's height makes it hard to conceal cannabis plants inside of pots because hemp grows close together and is usually grown in narrow rows. This causes the cannabis plant to stick out like a sore thumb. Not only that, but cannabis plants require a lot of sunlight which is difficult to get when hidden amongst hemp plants.

Another difference between hemp and cannabis is that cannabis must be grown in a warm and humid environment to be grown properly. Since hemp does not require the buds that cannabis does, hemp can be grown in almost any area where corn can grow.

Even though hemp is not required to flower to make CBD oil, it is still used to make the oil. It may even prove easier to make CBD oil out of hemp since you are not going to have to wait on the flowering process.

Hemp vs. Marijuana

You can make CBD oil out of hemp or marijuana. While CBD oil is legal as long as it's sourced from industrial hemp, you are going to end up giving up the THC levels when you get CBD oil that comes from hemp because hemp is low in THC levels and will grow in a sturdy stalk. Therefore, you are not going to get high when you consume CBD oil made from hemp.

But, CBD made from marijuana may or may not be legal for you depending on where you live. If you decide to use CBD with marijuana, look at the THC levels because they are vary based on what the dispensary does.

Hemp Oil vs. CBD Oil

It is important to understand the differences between Hemp Oil and CBD Oil but is also important to note that the oils get their names from the plants they are extracted from. Therefore, it is important to understand the similarities and differences between these plants before comparing the oils in detail.

Hemp Oil and CBD oil are both extracted from plants of the same species, Cannabis Sativa. But, there are a few differences between these plants which are important to note. These have been covered in detail at the beginning of the chapter. But, let us take a quick look at the differences before we look at the difference between the oils.

The cannabis plant, used to extract CBD oil, grows outward and has more buds and leaves while the hemp plant, used to extract Hemp oil, grows upward and has thick stalks. The cannabis plant is more like a shrub in the sense that it does not exceed more than five feet in height and needs a lot of space to grow. The hemp plant, on the other hand, can grow up to fifteen feet and can grow in small spaces. The significant difference between the plants is the proportion of cannabinoids or the chemical compounds found in the Cannabis sativa. There are close to 400 cannabinoids found in both hemp and cannabis of which the two most important cannabinoids are Cannabidiol (CBD) and tetrahydrocannabinol (TCH). These compounds are the most active cannabinoids in the plants and have been studied extensively by scientists and experts. It is very important to understand CBD and TCH so that one makes the right decision on which oil would need to be used.

Most cannabis smokers have either been high or have the feeling of being stoned because they smoke cannabis that has a higher concentration of TCH. It is because of this chemical that the drug has received negative reviews. CBD which is found in abundance in hemp is known for its relaxing properties and has been used since ancient times.

Oil that is extracted from the Cannabis sativa plant contains both the cannabinoids mentioned in different proportions. Cannabis contains only 10 percent of THC because of which the oil that is extracted from this is often used for recreation. However, hemp oil contains a higher proportion of CBD making it ideal to use for relaxing your mind and body.

Chapter 14

Rick Simpson Oil

We touched on Rick Simpson earlier, but in this chapter, we'll take a closer look at the man and how he made the oil using cannabis. It is easy to make Rick Simpson Oil at home using either hemp or cannabis (this method uses cannabis however you can use hemp as well). If you make the oil using hemp, it would not be the exact same oil made by Rick Simpson, but it would have the same effect on your body.

Rick Simpson, a Canadian engineer, used ingredients used to create cannabis oils (like hemp oil and CBD oil) and was able to cure himself of metastatic cancer in 2003. Since then, he has been attempting to educate people on how hemp oil is not as harmful as people believe it to be.

Simpson had resistance to his oil by Canadian authorities, government agencies, and big pharmaceutical companies as well as UN offices. This did not stop him though. Despite setbacks, he was able to treat 5,000 patients free of charge successfully using Hemp oil. These patients suffered from different diseases and conditions that they may have procured due to poor health choices or genetics.

In 2004, Rick Simpson got in touch with the Canadian Cancer Society about using hemp oil to cure cancer. However, the answer he got from the cancer society was anything but what he was looking for.

The society does not endorse or support medical products or dietary supplements... thanks for the information. Good luck in your work. – Canadian Cancer Society

It wasn't the reaction he was expecting.

Rick Simpson's Hemp oil (RSO) has been used not only for cancer but also for leukemia, arthritis, AIDS, HIV, Chron's disease, glaucoma, multiple sclerosis, diabetes, migraines, asthma, depression, osteoporosis, depress, burns, chronic pain, mutated cells, and to assist in regulating body weight.

When cannabis was administered for the first time, the oil was to be used for a period of 90 days. First, you'll start out with 3 doses daily for your first week. The serving size is somewhere around the size of a grain of rice. For the next 2 to 5 weeks you'll double your intake to 4 times a day. For the remaining weeks, you'll consume a gram of oil a day until all sixty grams are gone.

Those who have used RSO have said that it is bitter and tastes a little like chlorophyll. The best way to place the oil into your system without having to deal with the bitter taste is to place it on your lower gums and allow for your body to absorb it on its own.

You can make RSO out of cannabis. The process is similar to what we covered in chapter 10. You can follow the same instructions with a hemp plant, but obviously, you do not have to worry about THC since hemp contains a very small percentage of it.

You will first need to obtain an ounce of cannabis after it has been dried. After that, take the dry plant and place it into a plastic bucket. Next, cover it with a solvent of your choice and allow it to soak into the plant. To make sure the solvent soaks through the entire plant, break up the plant. You can do this while the cannabis bud is in the solvent. Stick to solvents like isopropyl, ether, naphtha, butane, or water. You'll need two gallons of solvent to extract the THC from your plant properly. This is only if you are using a pound if you are only using an ounce, you only need 500 milliliters.

After the solvent has been placed in the bucket, crush the cannabis plant with a spoon. As you crush the material, add more solvent to soak the material completely. Stir it for around three minutes so that the THC and CBD come out of the plant and settles into the liquid. Now, strain the cannabis out of your liquid by placing the solvent into a new bucket or bowl. You are only going to get around 80% of the oils out of the plant, and you'll need to repeat the process a time or two more to get the most out of the plant.

Discard the plant after the process and strain the liquid through a coffee filter. After that, fill up a rice cooker around 3/4 of the way full while heating it to high heat.

Note: make sure you're in a well-ventilated area! When you're doing this process, set up a fan and vent system so that the fumes you create can be evacuated away from your pot and you are not inhaling them. Wearing a mask to ensure you are not inhaling the fumes is advised. Also, avoid anything that could cause a spark such as a stove or a cigarette.

As the level decreases in your cooker, add more water, so that the solvent releases the oils that are stuck in it. These oils are your CBD and THC oils. Once you have burned about an inch of water out of the rice cooker, swirl the contents of your cooker until the solvent burns off completely. Don't use a heat that is over 290 °F.

Remove the pot from the burner yet again and pour it into a stainless-steel container. Now place that container inside of a dehydrator and allow a few hours for the water to evaporate from your oil. There should no longer be any surface activity on your oil so you should be able to use it right away. It's best to put the oil into a plastic syringe so that you can easily dispense with it after you've used it. Keep in mind that your oil will look a lot like grease when it has cooled.

Rick Simpson oil contains THC unlike CBD oil, and it gives you a euphoric feeling that CBD can't on its own. Also, CBD won't have the psychoactive element that Rick Simpson oil has. But, you can make Rick Simpson oil without THC if that is what you want. Just make sure you are using industrial hemp instead of the cannabis plant.

Unfortunately, companies and individuals will produce RSO that is abundant in THC and use Rick

Simpson's name to scam. It is best to either make the oil yourself as we've instructed in this book or buy it directly from Rick's website. If you see anything that has to do with the Phoenix Tears Foundation when you're searching for RSO, it is not from Rick Simpson as he does not have any association with this foundation.

Rick Simpson's official website is www.phoenixtears.ca where you can find more information about RSO and how it works as well as how to make it, buy it, and many other valuable pieces of information about how cannabis oil is good for you and how it can be used.

www.ingramcontent.com/pod-product-compliance
Lightning Source LLC
Chambersburg PA
CBHW070302230526
45470CB00002B/683